Temperature and You

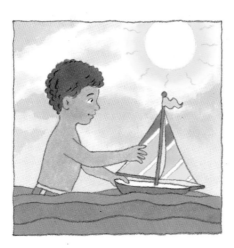
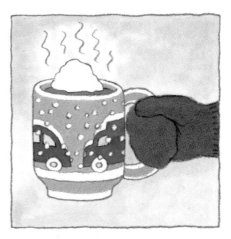
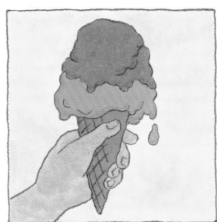
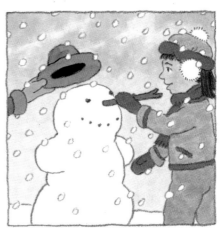

by Betsy and Giulio Maestro

Lodestar Books

Dutton   New York

Library of Congress Cataloging-in-Publication Data

Maestro, Betsy.
   Temperature and you / by Betsy and Giulio Maestro.
      p.   cm.
   Summary: Discusses what temperature is and how it is measured.
   ISBN 0-525-67271-0
   1. Temperature—Juvenile literature. 2. Thermometers and thermometry—Juvenile litera-
ture. [1. Temperature. 2. Thermometers and thermometry.] I. Maestro, Giulio. II. Title.
QC271.4.M34 1990   88-12934
536'.5—dc 19   CIP
                                                                                                AC

Published in the United States by Lodestar Books, an affiliate of Dutton Children's Books, a division of Penguin Books USA Inc.

Published simultaneously in Canada by Fitzhenry & Whiteside Limited, Toronto

Editor: Virginia Buckley   Designer: Richard Granald, LMD
Printed in Hong Kong by South China Printing Co.
First Edition   10 9 8 7 6 5 4 3 2 1

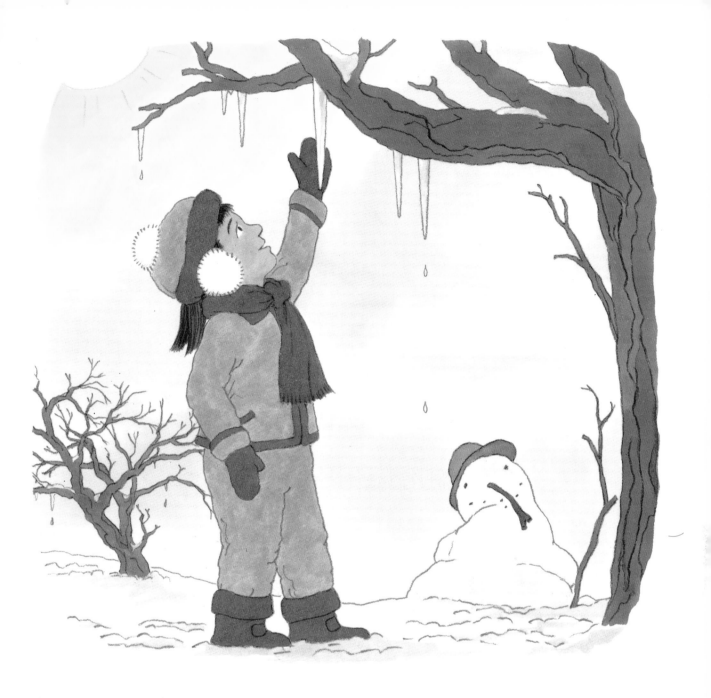

Hot and *cold, warm* and *cool* are words
that tell about temperature.
Temperature is how hot or cold something
or someone is.

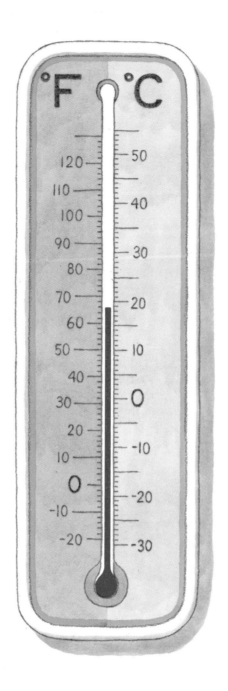

Temperature can be measured by a thermometer.
It shows you how hot or cold things are,
in numbers called degrees.

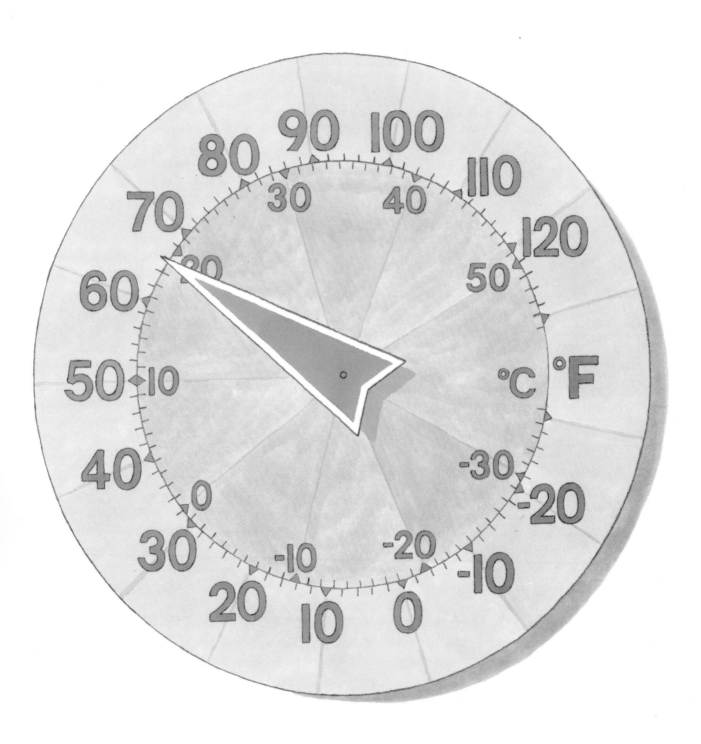

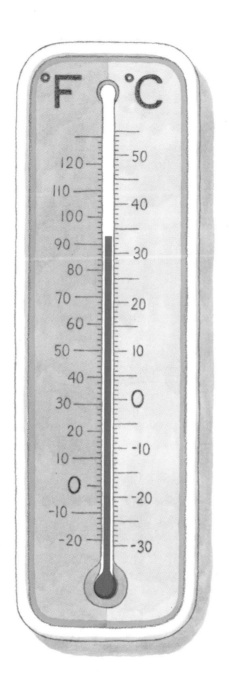

When the temperature is high, the red line in this thermometer goes up. This means that it is warm or hot. Outside on a hot summer day, the red line is always high or near the top.

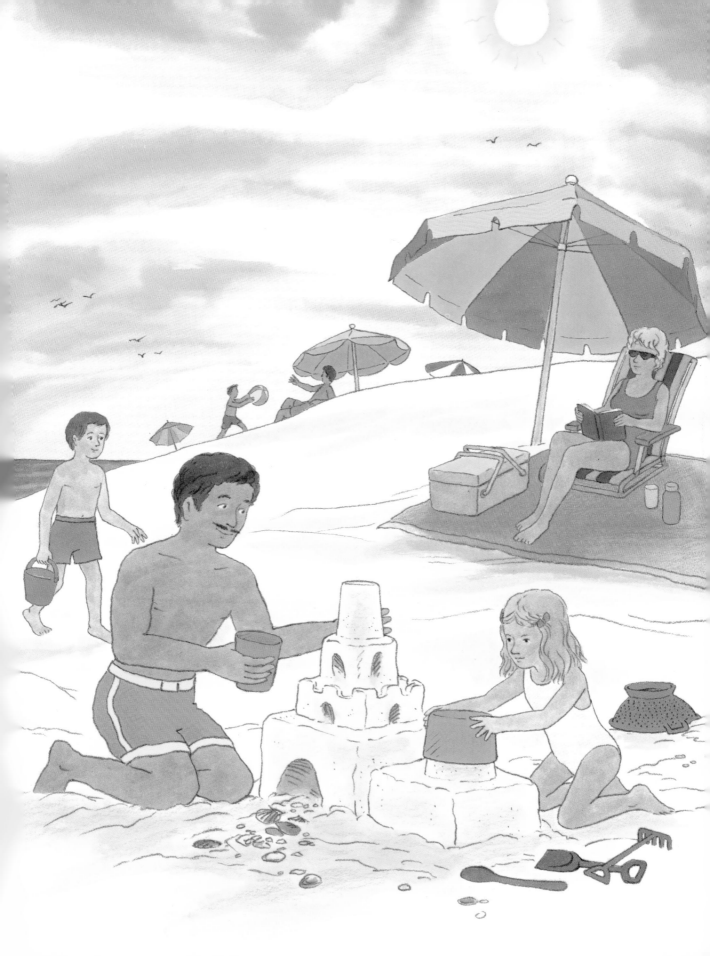

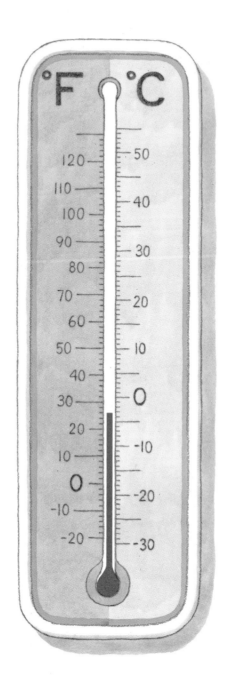

When the temperature is low, the red line in this thermometer goes down. This means that it is cool or cold. Outside on a cold winter day, the red line is usually low or near the bottom.

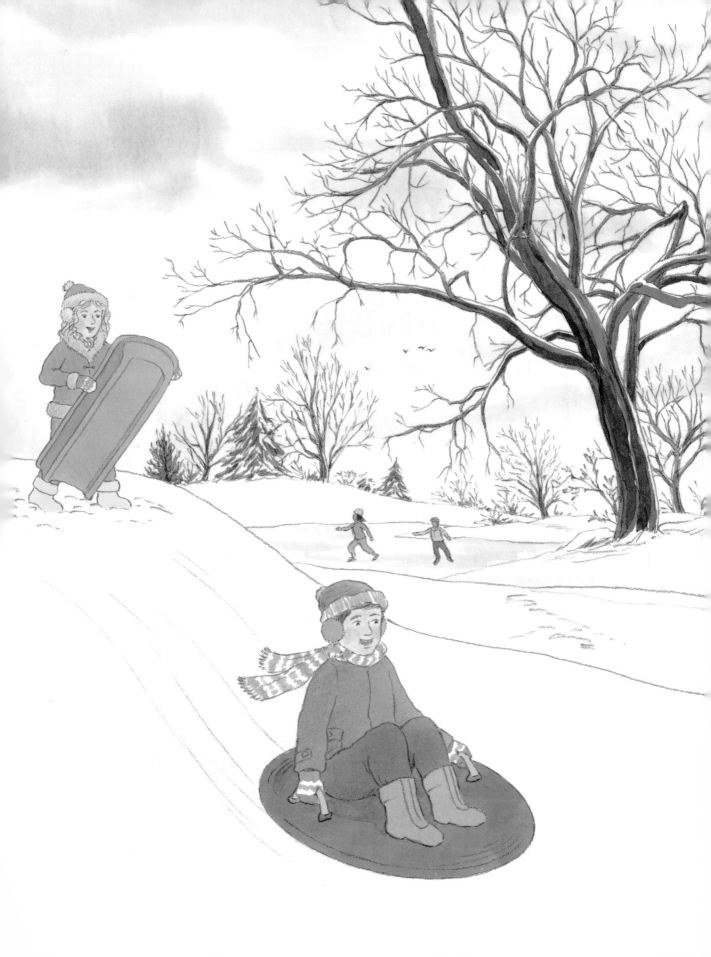

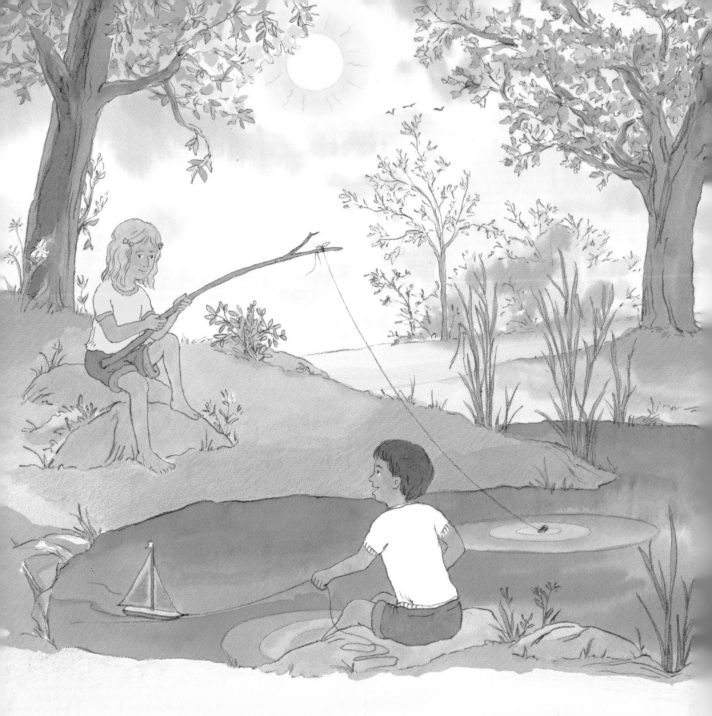

The temperature of the air changes because of the sun. The sun warms the air. In summer, there is a lot of sunshine, so the air is warm or hot. Temperatures go up.

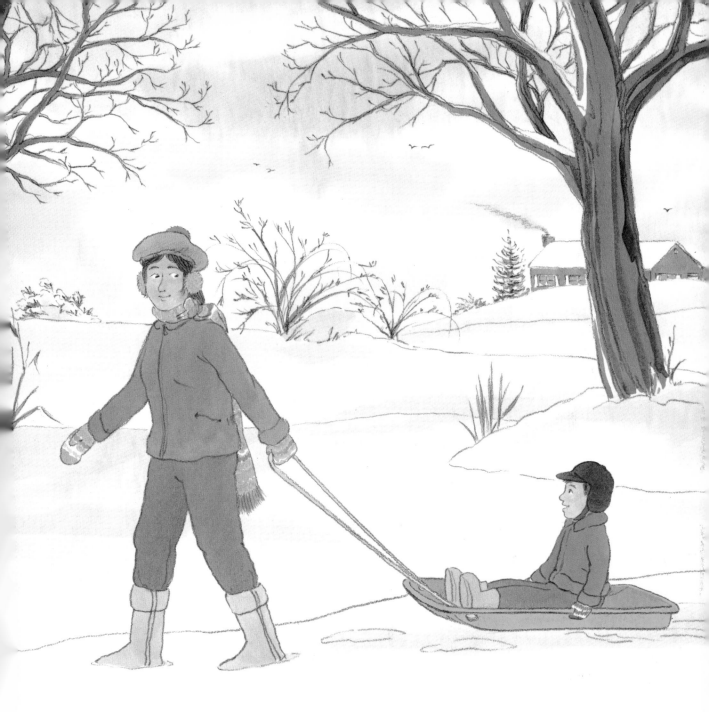

In winter, there is less sunshine, so the air is cool or cold. Temperatures go down.

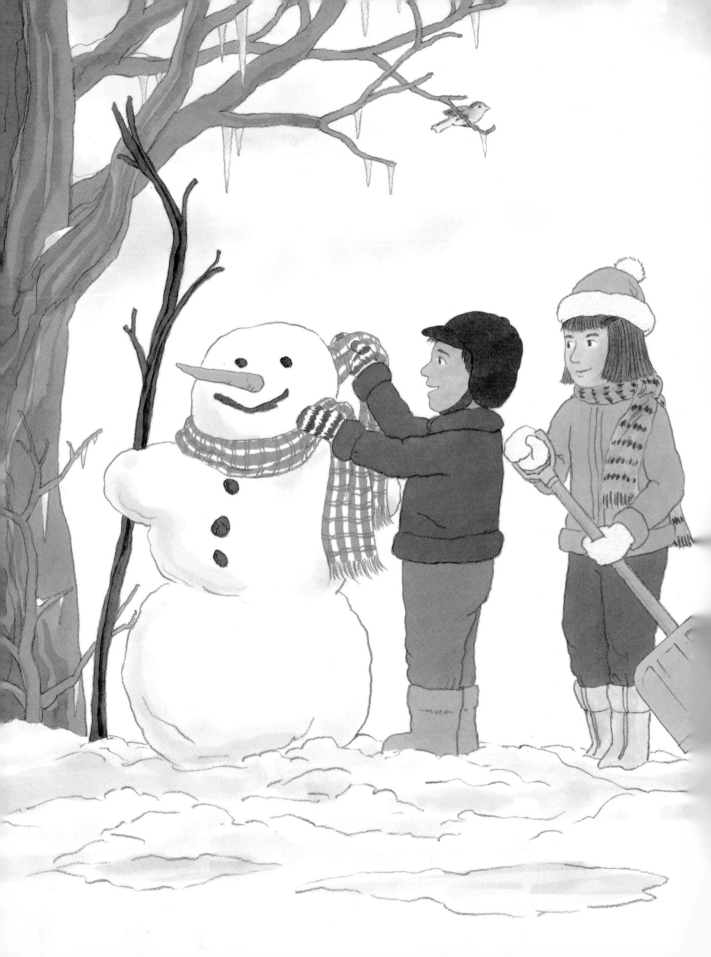

When the temperature is very cold, water freezes and becomes ice. If it gets warmer and the temperature goes up, the ice melts and becomes water again. Ice in your freezer stays frozen all the time.

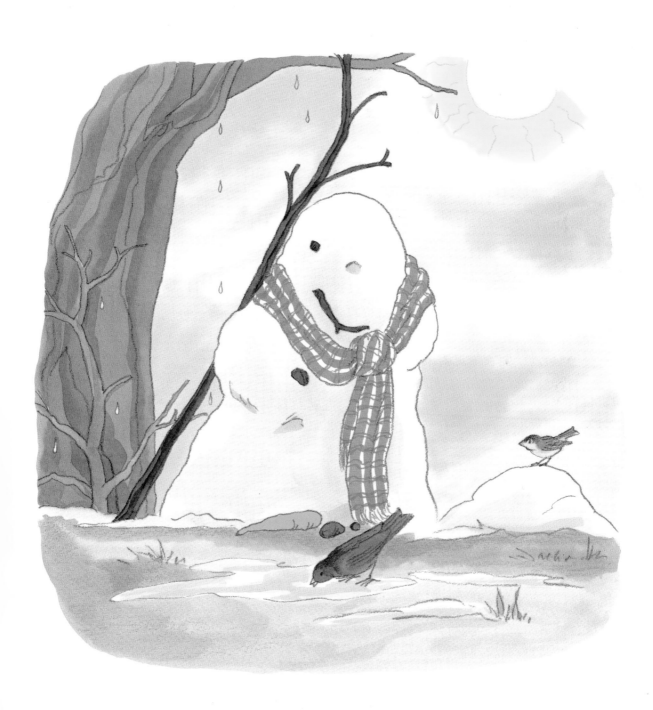

You cannot control the temperature outside. Inside your house, you can change the temperature to make it more comfortable. When it's cold, you can turn on the heat.

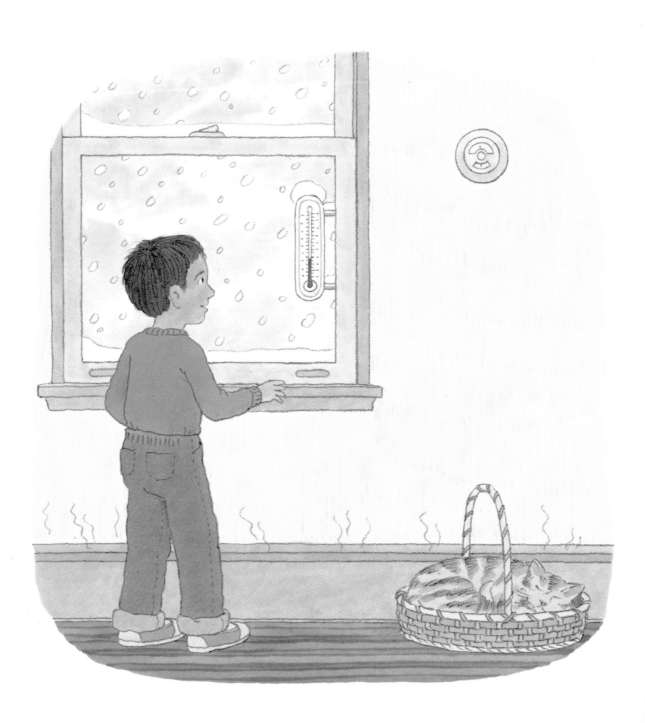

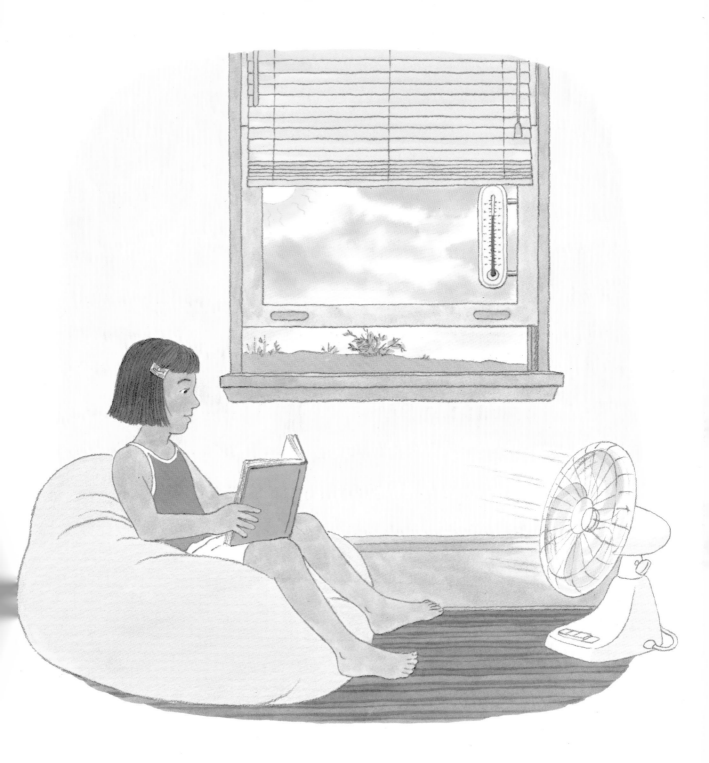

If it's too hot, you can use an air conditioner
or a fan.

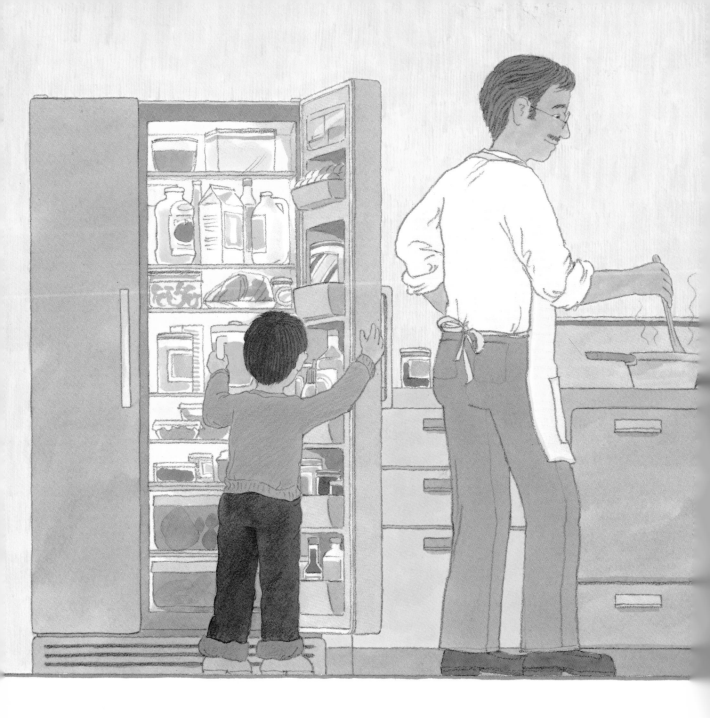

Heat and cold are used in your home in many helpful ways. The temperature inside the refrigerator stays cold all the time. Food stays fresh in cold temperatures.

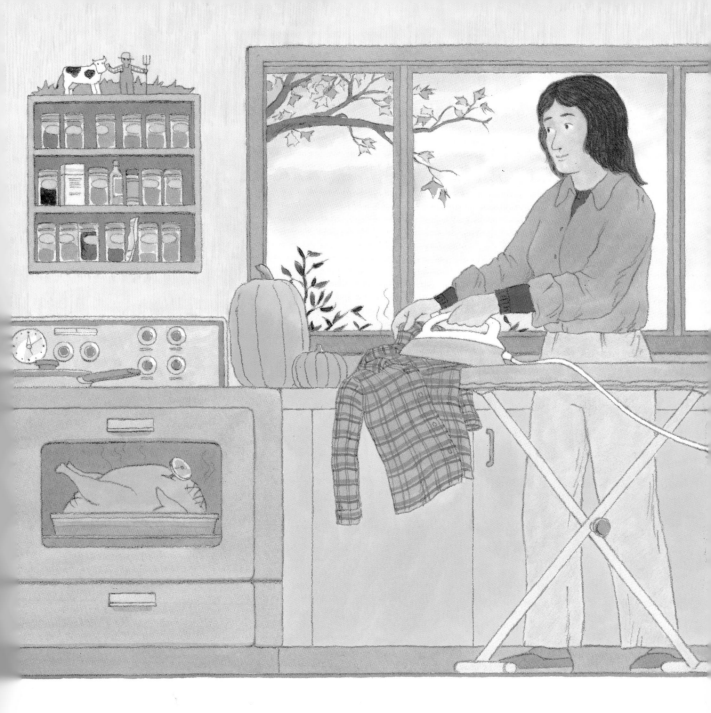

The heat of the oven cooks your food. A hot
iron smoothes wrinkles in your clothes.

The house you live in protects you from the cold and heat of outdoors. Your skin protects your body from very high or very low temperatures. Your body has its own temperature.

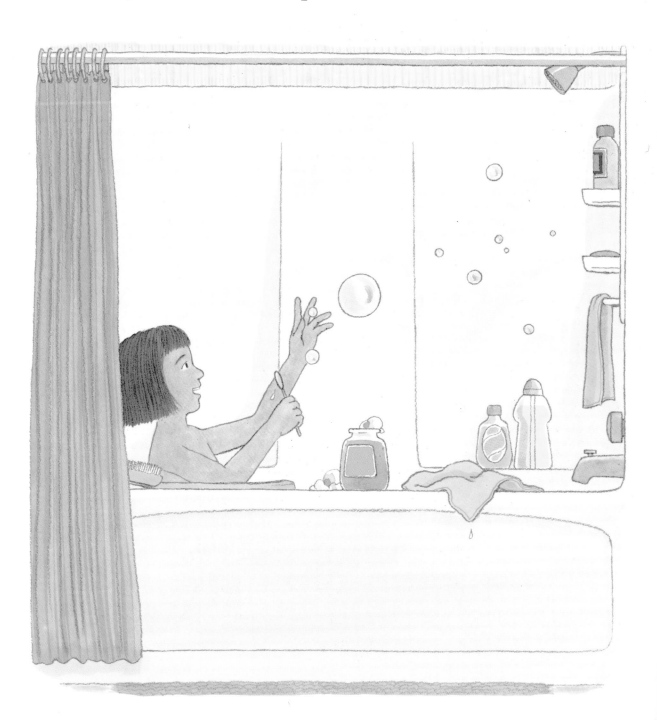

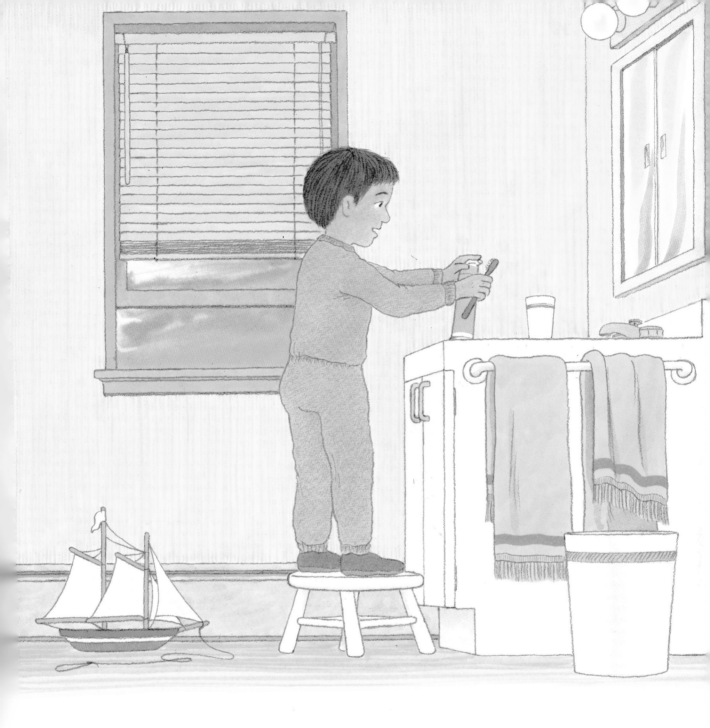

Skin helps keep your body at the right
temperature. It is a little like a blanket. Your
skin helps keep your body at about the same
temperature all the time.

Clothes help you stay warm or cool. If you wear many layers or very heavy clothing, your body heat stays next to you and keeps you warm.

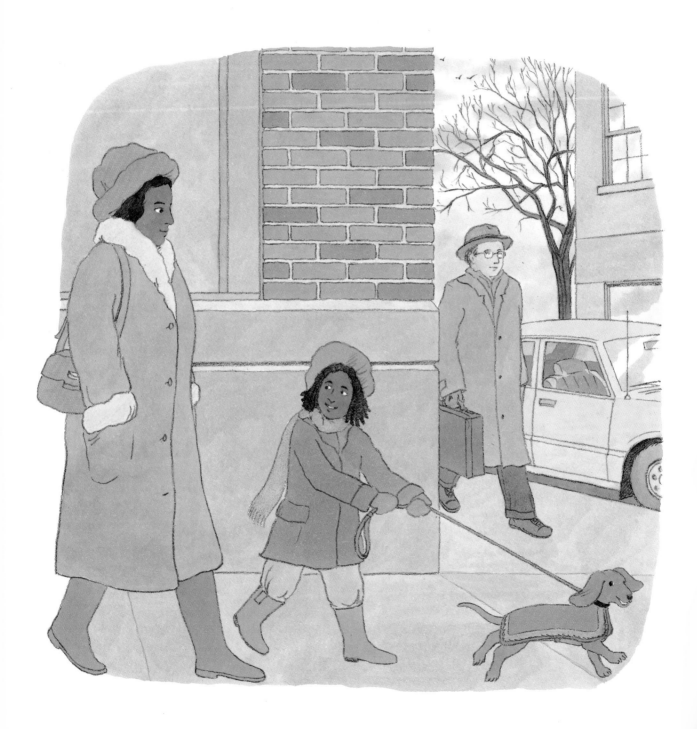

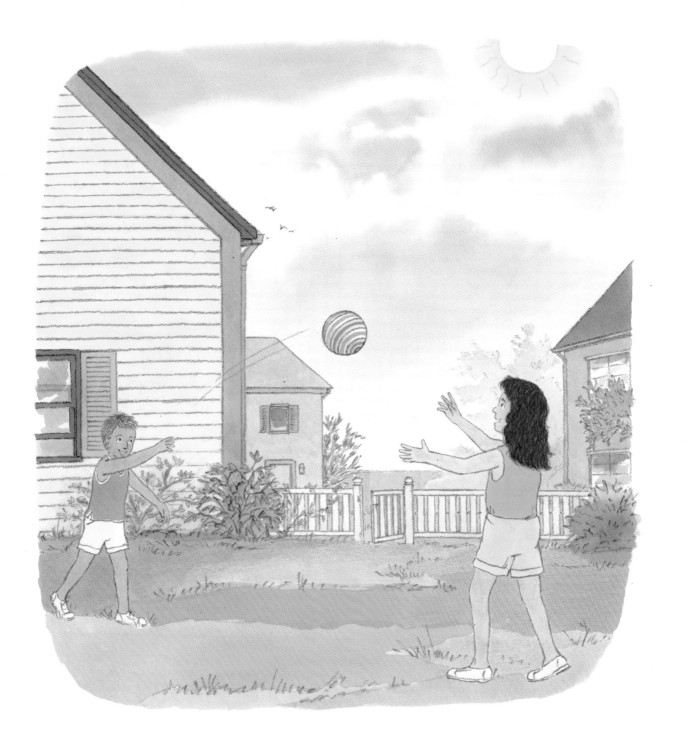

If you wear light, loose clothing, your body heat gets out and you feel cool.

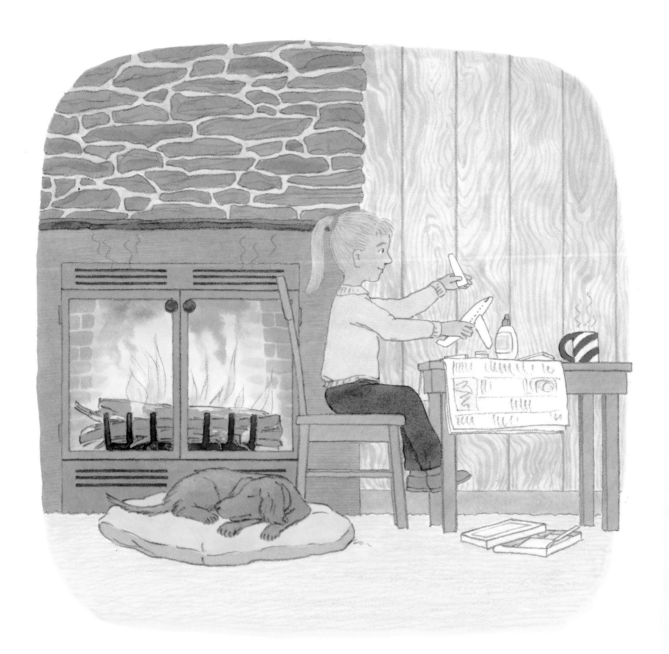

When the air is cold in winter and the temperature
is low, you can keep warm in many ways.
You can put on heavy clothes, drink warm cocoa,
and stay inside where fireplaces and furnaces
heat up the air.

When you go out, you can bundle up with lots of
extra clothing and move around a lot. Exercise makes
you feel warmer. If you get very cold, shivering
helps to warm you up.

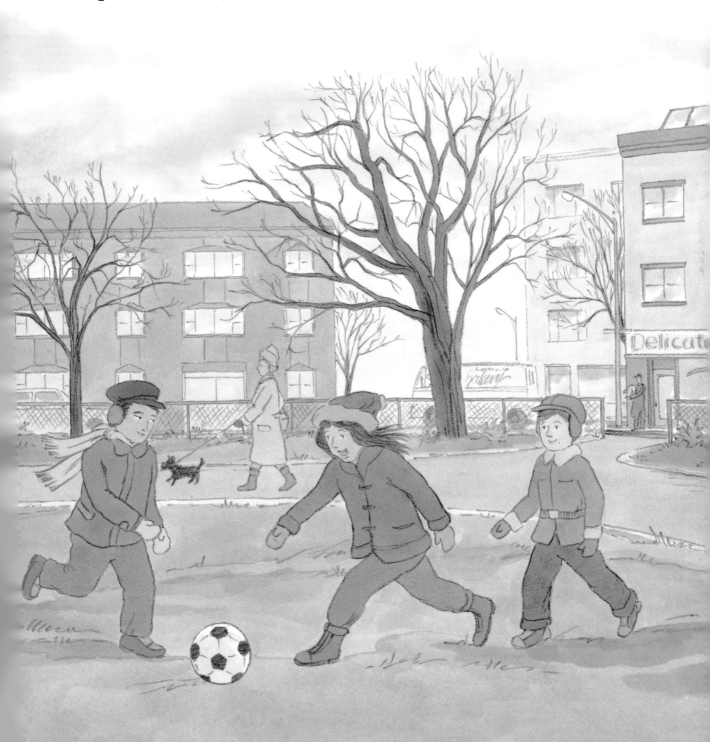

In summer, when the temperature is high, you can keep cool in many ways. You can wear thin, light clothing, have cold drinks, and stay inside rooms cooled by air conditioners or fans.

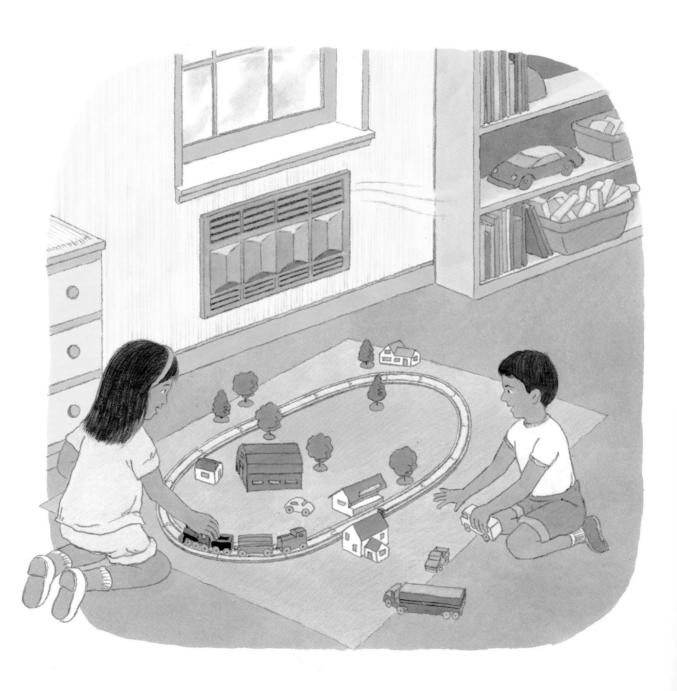

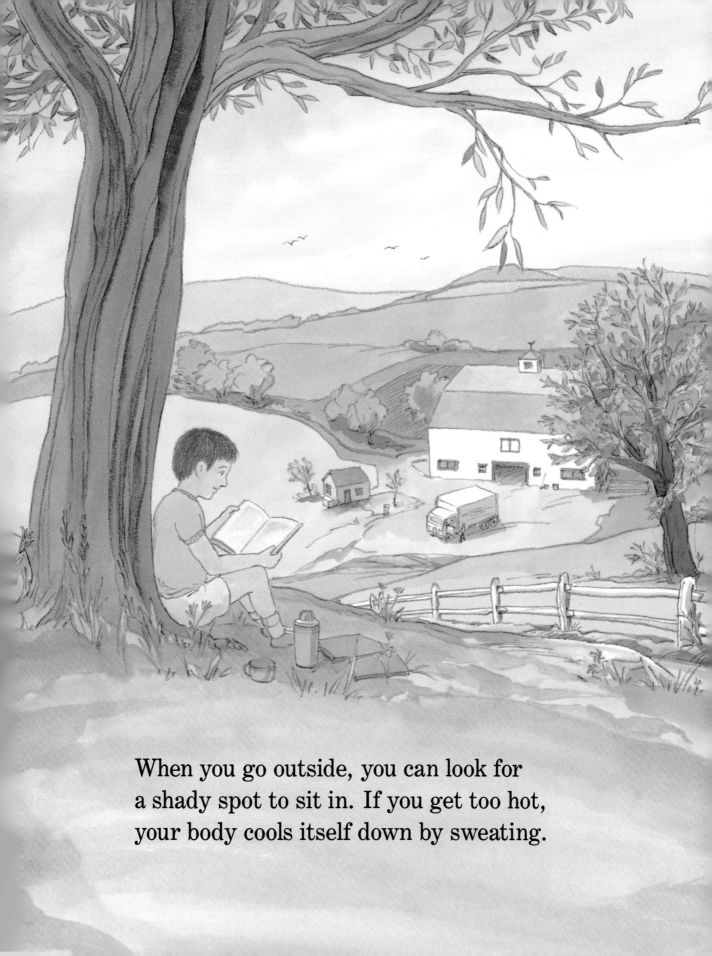

When you go outside, you can look for
a shady spot to sit in. If you get too hot,
your body cools itself down by sweating.

Your body temperature does not change with the weather or the seasons. But if you are ill, your body temperature may go up. When your body temperature is higher than it should be, you have a fever.

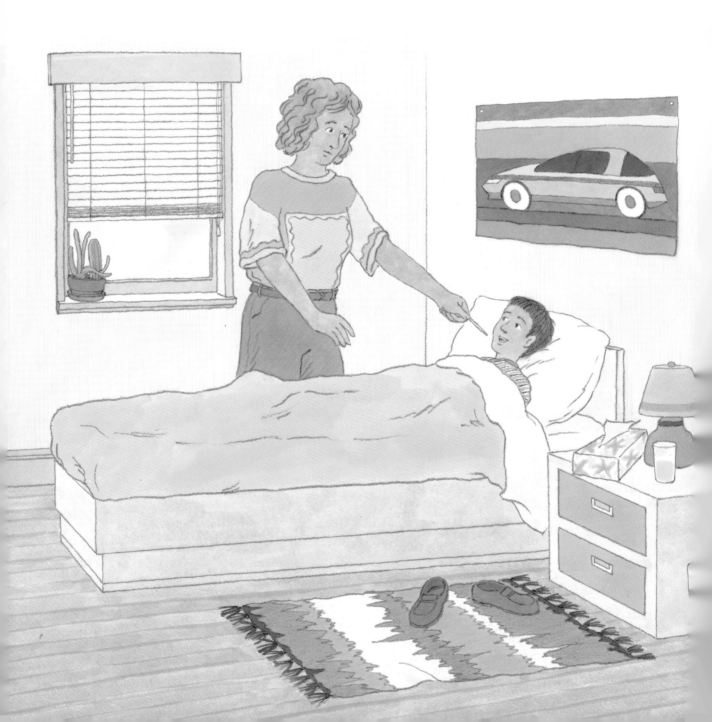

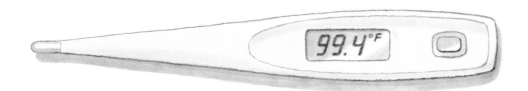

If you don't look well, or you feel hot, Mom or Dad will take your temperature with a fever thermometer. When they read the thermometer, they will know if you have a fever.

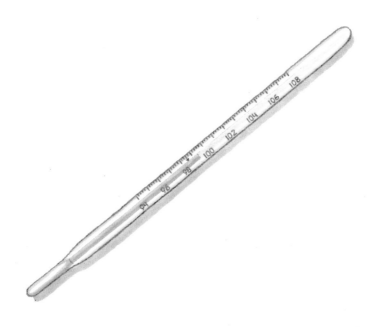

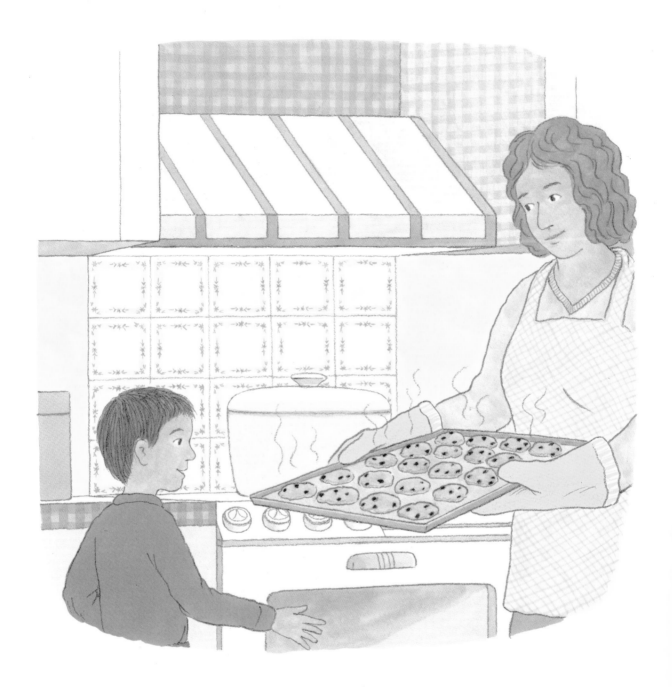

Temperature is important in your life. Knowing what the temperature is can help you decide how to dress, when to take food out of the oven, when to turn on the heat or open a window.

Sometimes you need a thermometer to tell you
exactly what the temperature is. Often you know
what the temperature is just by the way
you or something else feels.

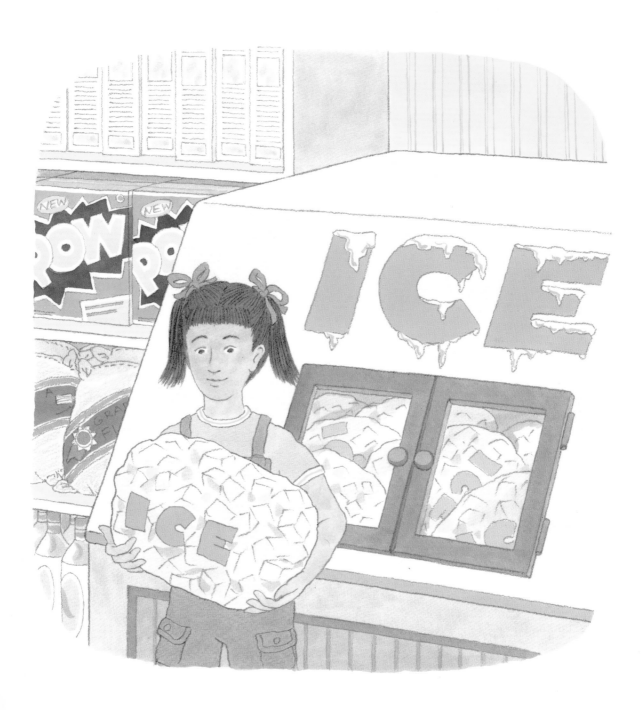

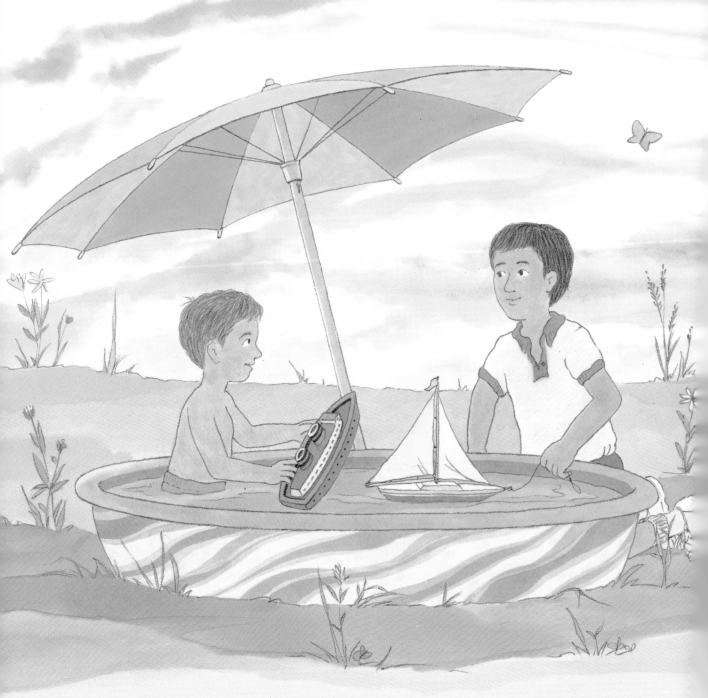

Everything has a temperature. Some things are hot and some are cold. You can learn to control the temperature of many things around you.

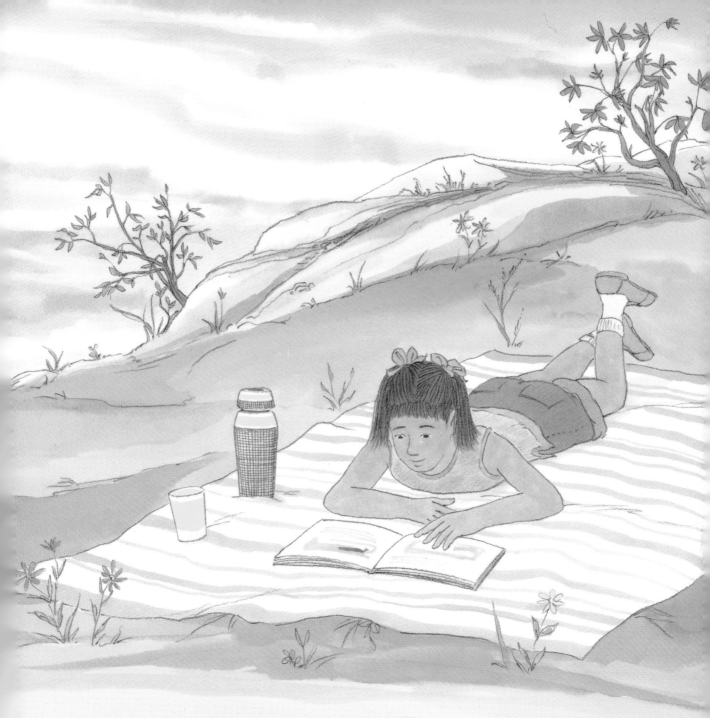

Even though you can't control the weather, you
can learn how to keep from getting too cold
or too hot. You feel most comfortable when the
temperature is just right for you.

Notes About Temperature

Body Temperature Normal human body temperature is about 98.6°F or 37°C.

Boiling Point The temperature at which a liquid boils. For water it is 212°F or 100°C.

Celsius A scale of temperature in degrees based on 100, with 0°C as the freezing point and 100°C as the boiling point. Same as centigrade.

Fahrenheit A scale of temperature in degrees based on 32°F as the freezing point and 212°F as the boiling point.

Freezing Point The temperature at which a liquid freezes. For water it is 32°F or 0°C.

Shivering Shaking or trembling from cold; a process by which the body automatically warms itself. The movement of so many muscles generates more body heat.

Sweating Release of moisture from the pores on the skin, usually when the body is overheated. This liquid, called sweat, is made up of water and chemicals and is produced by the sweat glands. As the sweat comes through the pores all over the body, it evaporates and the body cools. Body heat is released into the air through evaporation.

536
MAE

Maestro, Betsy

Temperature and you

$13.95